Pegan Diet

An Indispensable Handbook For Navigating The Path To
A Healthier Lifestyle: Recommended Dietary Choices And
Foods To Steer Clear Of

*(A Comprehensive Collection Of Proven And Reliable
Recipes)*

Vladimir Cousineau

TABLE OF CONTENT

Introduction

We reside in an expeditious society that displays a reluctance to accommodate delays for anyone. If you are unable to maintain pace, you will be surpassed and left behind. As a result, numerous individuals are inclined to make various sacrifices in their lives. This is mostly time. This represents an opportunity to devote their time to spending quality moments with their loved ones, unwinding, or preparing a nutritious and balanced meal. Occasionally indulging in meals commonly referred to as "junk food" is permissible, however, when it becomes a regular habit due to a lack of time for consuming healthier alternatives, a concerning issue arises.

Numerous varieties of unhealthy food, including instant meals, undergo extensive processing, possess minimal nutritional content, and contain significant amounts of preservatives and sodium. In minimal quantities, this issue is scarcely consequential, yet contemporary individuals are increasingly relying on these meals as their fundamental sustenance. Numerous individuals assert that they engage in this activity due to its expediency and convenience; however, can this notion truly be substantiated?

According to Health24 (2019), the year 2017 witnessed an alarming figure of 11 million fatalities attributed to subpar dietary practices. Heart disease was the predominant cause of mortality, accounting for 10 million deaths. Subsequently, individuals succumbed to cancer, followed by type 2 diabetes, according to the Cleveland Clinic's report in 2019. The total fatality count surpassed the combined number of individuals who succumbed to high blood pressure or tobacco consumption in the corresponding year. These fatalities accounted for 22% of the total number of deaths among adults that were documented. That constitutes approximately 20 percent of the population. Consider the following: The mortality rate of individuals not consuming a balanced diet reached an alarming figure of one in five. While it may be convenient to attribute blame solely to junk food, regrettably, it is not the sole perpetrator.

Despite the abundance of nutritious food options available, individuals persist in opting for detrimental dietary choices that can compromise their overall well-being. Individuals often gravitate towards food options that exhibit elevated sodium levels, undergo extensive processing, lack sufficient fiber content, and feature unhealthy fats such as artificial trans fats. This inclination is primarily driven by the palatability of such foods as well as their affordability and widespread availability. These imbalanced diets may temporarily satiate hunger, but they fail to provide the essential nutrients required for the body to operate optimally, especially considering the demanding lifestyle that many individuals embrace.

An imbalanced diet can potentially result in fatal outcomes, such as heart disease, diabetes, and cancer. However, it is worth noting that there are various other ailments that can be linked to this condition. Eating disorders, dental caries, excessive weight, depressive symptoms, and even the development of osteoporosis are associated with a suboptimal dietary pattern, to provide a limited list of examples.

According to a comprehensive analysis conducted by the Cleveland Clinic in 2019, the United States occupied the 45th position among 195 countries in terms of mortality due to suboptimal dietary decisions over the period spanning from 1990 to 2017. In order to mitigate the risk of these diseases and premature mortality, individuals must reclaim control over their time and lives. Contrary to popular belief, it is not as challenging as commonly perceived. Before any modifications can be implemented, it is imperative to establish a comprehensive comprehension of both detrimental lifestyle patterns and an unhealthy dietary regimen. One of the initial measures to take is to forgo highly processed commodities in exchange for whole foods. Wholefood products encompass the essential dietary fiber required for maintaining a healthy gastrointestinal system, while also exerting a decelerating effect on the release of energy derived from the glucose content present in the food. Exert the endeavor to substitute unhealthy snacks with homemade meals, or preferably minimally processed meals, which ought to comprise the majority of one's dietary intake.

A significant number of contemporary dietary approaches advocate for an increased consumption of plant-based foods in lieu of animal products, driven by factors encompassing ethical considerations, environmental concerns, as well as improvements in health. It is strongly recommended to consume at least two servings of fruit and five servings of vegetables, as these food groups provide numerous essential nutrients that contribute to promoting overall physical well-being. Through the consumption of fewer animal-derived dietary products, individuals can effectively reduce their intake of saturated fats and cholesterol.

Nonetheless, what criteria should be taken into consideration when selecting a suitable dietary plan for oneself? There exists a diverse spectrum ranging from highly committed vegans to entirely devoted carnivores. Which option would you prefer? Might I propose a solution that strikes a balance between endorsing sustainable dietary practices, providing essential nutrients, and advocating for a predominantly plant-centered eating pattern? The pegan diet satisfies all the criteria. This dietary regimen necessitates the consumption of a substantial portion of fresh produce, primarily comprising fruits and vegetables, while not imposing strict veganism upon individuals. Despite its limitations, the dietary regimen does advocate modest consumption of meat in order to ensure a comprehensive intake of essential nutrients predominantly found in animal-derived sources.

While there exist a few limitations to the diet, similar to other dietary plans, the primary constraint entails eliminating all processed foods and opting for whole foods instead. This can be astonishingly uncomplicated when you dedicate the necessary time to contemplate alternative options for your existing dietary regimen. One should consider substituting fruit juice with whole fruits and opting for water to satisfy thirst, given the simplicity of this change.

Through acquiring The Pegan Diet: The Simple and Fast Way to Sustain Optimal Health—Effortless and Flavorful Recipes Prepared Within 30 Minutes, one will develop an appreciation for the significance of a holistic dietary approach that entails limitations on specific food items known to elevate blood sugar levels and instigate inflammation. Uncover the advantages of adhering to a pegan diet, while simultaneously acquiring knowledge regarding the optimal food choices for this diet, as well as those that should be permanently disregarded.

One of the foremost challenges encountered by individuals while transitioning to a new dietary regimen is the arduous task of discerning the requisite preparations and cooking methods necessary to adhere to the prescribed diet. This has been streamlined for your convenience through a four-week dietary plan that enables you to conveniently procure the precise items required for each week of your diet. Furthermore, this book encompasses a wide range of recipes that cater to various dietary requirements, encompassing main meals, beverages, snacks, and desserts, specifically tailored to individuals following the pegan diet. Given these circumstances, the most arduous aspect of transitioning to a pegan diet will entail perusing a meticulously compiled inventory of groceries, deliberating over which culinary creation to embark upon initially.

Ensure that you do not allow your physical well-being to deteriorate, especially when you currently possess the opportunity to rectify your dietary habits. Do not hold the belief that this task can be accomplished upon identification of an illness. It is recommended that you make a committed endeavor to adopt a new dietary regimen today, as it has the potential to forestall the onset of a debilitating ailment within your body. Proceed by flipping the page to commence.

Chapter 1: The Diet

A nutritious diet is crucial for maintaining optimal physical well-being, as food encompasses more than mere sustenance. Frequently, individuals express the sentiment that your dietary choices dictate your physical well-being. This statement is not strictly literal, yet it does possess an element of veracity. The sustenance we consume serves a purpose beyond mere energy transportation. The nutrients derived from our dietary intake undergo a process of decomposition within the body, serving various essential functions such as the development of muscular tissues (proteins), the generation of energy (carbohydrates), and the formation of hormones (fats), to outline only the macronutrients and a few of their respective roles.

A proper or balanced diet additionally plays a role in enhancing your holistic health, given that an assortment of essential minerals, vitamins, and antioxidants collectively contribute to your overall well-being. By prioritizing self-care and focusing on internal wellness, individuals can actively shield themselves against noncommunicable ailments including specific forms of cancer, type 2 diabetes, obesity, and mitigate the chances of developing cardiovascular disorders. One can attain this objective by adhering to a nutritionally balanced diet comprising primarily of fresh and diverse food choices, while concurrently reducing the intake of sugar, salt, and saturated fats, and completely eliminating the consumption of trans fats and highly refined processed foods.

There exists a plethora of dietary regimens presently accessible on a global scale, aiding diverse individuals in achieving their desired healthier body weights and enhancing their overall well-being, thereby mitigating the likelihood of various severe ailments that are commonly linked to an inadequate dietary lifestyle.

What Does the Pegan Diet Method Entail?

The pegan diet is an amalgamation of two firmly established dietary approaches, namely the vegan diet and the paleo diet. Individually, these dietary regimens can pose challenges in terms of sustainability; however, when combined, they become slightly more manageable. From the perspective of the vegan aspect of this dietary regimen, it is highly recommended to incorporate a diverse assortment of fresh fruits and vegetables into your meals on a frequent basis. A significant portion amounting up to 75% of your daily dietary intake ought to be comprised of this particular category of food. These products are most suitable when sourced from organic origins. While it is advisable to primarily derive nutrition from plant-based sources, it is essential to acknowledge certain constraints regarding the selection of plant varieties. It is advisable to refrain from consuming plant-based food items that possess both a high glycemic index and a high gluten content, as such foods exert a greater influence on blood sugar levels and have the potential to promote inflammation.

In adherence to the paleolithic aspect of this dietary regimen, it is permissible to incorporate various animal-derived goods into one's culinary choices, albeit not exceeding a 25% proportion of the overall diet. Moreover, it is paramount that such animal products are procured through ethical means, ensuring that the animals were fed a natural grass-based diet and were raised in pastures. Fish is permissible within the dietary plan, although it is advisable to opt for fish varieties with minimal mercury content, such as wild salmon and sardines.

Why the Pegan Diet?

This dietary regimen not only promotes personal well-being but also contributes positively to environmental sustainability. Traditional agriculture practices have the potential to introduce harmful substances, such as pesticides, herbicides, and other undesirable components, into the immediate environment. Additionally, the transportation of goods associated with conventional farming can lead to increased carbon emissions, creating a larger ecological footprint. Furthermore, it can assist in the avoidance of the consumption of genetically modified organisms (GMOs) for which insufficient long-term studies have been conducted to ascertain the potential consequences of regular and prolonged ingestion. Additionally, the consumption of organic produce and products not only serves to support the expansion of local enterprises, but further contributes to the preservation of economic resources within the community.

There are numerous health advantages associated with adhering to this diet as it involves the elimination of heavily processed foods, sugar, unhealthy fats, the majority of grain and legume consumption, and a moderate intake of meat. The dietary regimen has the objective of reducing inflammation, regulating blood sugar levels, promoting a wholesome way of living, and enhancing overall well-being.

Benefits of the Diet

This diet is relatively nascent, and comprehensive scientific investigations regarding the advantages of this dietary approach are still lacking. Nevertheless, this diet encompasses numerous advantages stemming from the adoption of clean eating principles. By increasing your consumption of a diverse range of fruits and vegetables, you are effectively introducing various essential minerals and vitamins into your body. These nutrients play a pivotal role in safeguarding against various illnesses and ailments. This particular type of food is additionally abundant in dietary fiber, which facilitates the gradual release of sugar and serves as a prebiotic for intestinal microflora. Moreover, it contains a significant amount of antioxidants that effectively combat the detrimental effects of oxidative stress on your body. Plant-based diets have previously demonstrated efficacy in promoting weight loss and reducing elevated levels of harmful cholesterol to more desirable ranges. Certain plant-based foods should be avoided due to their impact on blood sugar levels.

By completely eliminating trans fats and reducing the consumption of saturated fats, you can significantly decrease the likelihood of experiencing cardiovascular complications. Reducing the intake of animal products can additionally result in a decrease in the consumption of "undesirable" cholesterol. This diet does not impose as many limitations as numerous others, as it permits a considerable variety of food items and does not impose constraints on calorie intake or specific eating times. By opting to consume organic food, you are actively promoting the environmentally sustainable practices that benefit the collective welfare of society. In general, adopting a diet consisting of nutritious food options will enhance the overall quality of your dietary intake, ultimately promoting improved health and well-being for yourself. This dietary regimen is well-suited for individuals with gluten and dairy sensitivities, or those seeking an alternative means to regulate their blood sugar levels via nutritional choices.

"The Distinctions Between The Pegan Diet And Other Prominent Dietary Approaches

The Pegan diet has emerged as a highly sophisticated dietary regimen that has gained significant acclaim. Allow me to present an alternative approach wherein it accumulates in opposition to conventional dietary patterns.

Paleo

This dietary regimen focuses on high-quality animal products such as meat, fish, and eggs, in addition to fats, vegetables, fruits, nuts, and seeds. The Paleo diet excludes grains, dairy, vegetables, sugar, and processed food. Given that pegan has derived partially from paleo, there exist several resemblances, albeit with notable distinctions being that pegan permits specific types of grains, legumes, vegetables, and indigenous dairy.

Veggie Lover

The second aspect that incited the emergence of pegan, which pertains to a plant-based diet, abstains from all animal products or anything deriving from the maternal source. It revolves around the consumption of plant-derived food items, whilst deliberately eschewing any products derived from animals. The Pegan diet advocates for the conscious selection of environmentally friendly and ethically sourced foods, resembling the principles of veganism. However, it allows for the inclusion of limited quantities of meat and other animal products. Both adherents to plant-based diets and practitioners of the pegan lifestyle prioritize the significance of vegetables and organic produce.

Vegan

Compared to individuals who strictly adhere to a plant-based diet, there exist multiple variations of vegetarianism. While certain individuals permit the consumption of fish and eggs, there are others who permit the consumption of dairy products. Vegan consumers may find a strong alignment with the dietary principles of peganism, which involves consuming limited quantities of meat and animal products.

Keto

The Ketogenic diet primarily focuses on the consumption of a restricted quantity of carbohydrates, while emphasizing a substantive intake of fats and moderate levels of protein. The ketogenic diet consists of a relatively lower proportion of vegetables and fruits, as both of these food groups naturally contain carbohydrates. Conversely, it tends to be comparatively higher in fat and animal-based protein content when compared to the Pegan diet. Although it is technically possible to adhere to a paleo-keto lifestyle, incorporating a Pegan diet alongside a ketogenic eating pattern proves to be challenging due to the inherent difficulty associated with composing a plate predominantly consisting of 75% vegetables and fruits.

DASH

The DASH diet, an acronym for Dietary Approaches to Stopping Hypertension, is commonly employed in cases where there is elevated cholesterol, increased risk of coronary disease, or the presence of diabetes. The foundation of DASH revolves around the principle of maintaining sodium levels that are notably lower than those found in the typical American diet, while emphasizing the inclusion of ample quantities of vegetables, fruits, whole grains, and low-fat dairy products. DASH recommends consuming a daily intake of 6 to 8 servings of grains. It also places emphasis on the consumption of lean meats, poultry, and fish while limiting the intake of fats and oils to two servings per day. DASH and pegan exhibit opposing characteristics in relation to certain notable variables. Pegan diet advocates for the moderate integration of grains, whereas the DASH diet emphasizes the incorporation of grains due to their essential nutritional composition. The DASH diet regimen includes monitoring sodium intake and encourages the consumption of low-fat dairy products, while the pegan diet disregards the role of sodium when processed food options are eliminated. Pegan comprehensively impacts dairy products derived from cow's milk.

Mediterranean Diet

The Mediterranean diet similarly prioritizes cardiovascular well-being and underscores several comparable principles as the Pegan diet. Both advocate for increased consumption of vegetables, incorporating vegetable oil, and maintaining regular fish intake. However, starting from that period, they exhibit differences. The Mediterranean diet promotes the consumption of vegetable oils, reduced sodium intake, increased consumption of whole grains, and imposes strict limitations on meat consumption to only a few times per month. The core focus of the Pegan diet lies in the utilization of oils, with the exception of individuals adhering to a vegetable-based lifestyle and limited to consumption of whole grains. While it is not proven that meat must be the most consumed food, the pegan diet leans towards moderate consumption of high-quality meat. Nevertheless, the Mediterranean dietary pattern actively reduces the consumption of meat.

Comprehensive Guidelines for the Efficient and Secure Implementation of a Pegan Program to Optimize Weight Loss

Whenever you embark upon a new dietary regimen, it is always prudent to consult with your physician. Prior to initiating a dietary transition, it is highly advisable to undergo a comprehensive blood analysis, specifically focusing on indicators of inflammation, lipid levels, glucose, insulin, and beyond. This meticulous assessment will enable you to monitor your progress in achieving desired outcomes and enhancing your overall health through dietary modifications. The reduction of pounds on the scale should not be considered as the sole indicators of one's overall well-being. In certain instances, improvements in other markers of well-being may precede the commencement of weight loss.

According to Hyman, this relates to customizing the approach rather than following a standardized system. Certain aspects of the Pegan diet may not be suitable for individuals who suffer from diabetes or other medical conditions. The location serves as a beneficial setting for engaging in group check-ins with your clinical team, which can establish the foundation for your progress. Over time, your nutritional needs may also undergo alteration. Pegan typically demonstrates a notable degree of flexibility, allowing for substantial opportunities for customization within its underlying foundations.

Specifically, pegan consumption does not revolve around adversity or prohibition, but rather focuses on sustenance and conscientiousness. Maintaining a considerable distance from handled and sweet food sources holds significant importance— nonetheless, this does not imply a desire to experience deprivation. Within the pages of this book, you will discover a plethora of techniques for crafting divine meals, appetizers, and even desserts utilizing pegan-friendly ingredients.

Comprehensive Guidelines for Initiating a Pegan Diet

Initiating a Pegan diet can be undertaken through several distinct approaches. This book provides over 125 comprehensive strategies to initiate your journey, including a meticulously crafted meal plan that spans an entire month. If the need arises for you to make a significant decision, it would be advisable to commence with the consideration of the dinner plan. However, in addition, you will also emphasize the strategies outlined in this book to acquire knowledge about the Pegan diet for a duration of two to four weeks in order to experiment with this novel approach to nourishment. You will soon realize that the plans are easy to comprehend and execute. Nevertheless, these food items possess a delightful taste without any lingering aftertaste reminiscent of tedious, restrictive dietary consumption.

Pegan is frequently a practice that one simply adheres to. Alternatively, you may consider implementing the 80/20 approach, wherein the majority of your dietary choices conform to the pegan guidelines throughout the week, and allowing yourself more culinary freedom on the weekends. The advantages of adhering solely to the pegan diet are not limited to only following the prescribed guidelines; rather, the more meals you align with this dietary approach, the greater the benefits you will experience.

If the idea of immediately diving into a month-long meal plan seems overwhelming, consider incorporating one pegan day per week and gradually progress towards implementing this dietary regimen for all seven days. Once you become well-acquainted with the dietary guidelines and attune yourself to them, you will no longer exert excessive mental effort, as you will have the opportunity to seamlessly incorporate them into your everyday routine. Constituting a supportive community of individuals as an supplementary approach to dining can also enhance success rates and consequently yield significant satisfaction.

In the event that your partner or relatives are not adhering to the Pegan diet alongside you, it would be beneficial to seek a companion to accompany you. You will engage in a reciprocal arrangement, where meals will be exchanged and culinary insights on food preparation and preferred formulas will be shared. This mutual support will serve as a source of motivation to persevere in your culinary endeavors.

The Pegan diet is considered to be safe and beneficial for individuals, including pregnant and lactating women, due to its lack of calorie restrictions. While excessive promotion of personal endorsement from medical professionals may dominate, pegan stands out as a reliable option due to its inclusive nature, as it encompasses a wide variety of unprocessed, nutrient-rich foods.

Green Beans, Four Ways

Ingredients:

- .1 cup mixed sliced mushrooms
- ¼ cup packaged fried onions
- ¼ cup toasted slivered almonds
- .2 teaspoons sesame oil over
- .1 tablespoon toasted sesame seeds
- 1 cup water
- .4 pounds green beans, trimmed
- .Salt and pepper
- .2 teaspoons extra-virgin olive oil
- .2 tablespoons finely grated parmesan cheese

Directions:

1. Place the water into the pressure cooker vessel. Insert a liner into the cooking appliance. Please position the beans within the liner insert.

2. Securely close the lid and adjust the timer to a duration of 2 minutes under high tension. When the clock ceases to function, promptly alleviate the pressure and reveal the lid. Transfer the beans to a serving bowl utilizing appropriate utensils.

3. "Enhance the flavor of the beans using any of the following seasoning options:

4. Coat the beans evenly by combining them with salt, pepper, 2 teaspoons of extra-virgin olive oil, and 2 tablespoons of finely ground Parmesan cheese.

5. Apply a measure of one tablespoon of unsalted spread onto the heated beans, then season with salt and pepper. Utilize culinary implements to enhance dispersion and envelopment of the

beans. Gently scatter ¼ cup of almonds that have been toasted and broken into fragments.

6. Pour 2 teaspoons of sesame oil evenly onto the beans and season with an appropriate amount of salt and pepper. Use the utensils to toss the beans and ensure they are coated with the oil. Evenly distribute the toasted sesame seeds, one tablespoon in quantity, onto the uppermost layer of the beans.

7. Sautee one cup of mixed diced mushrooms in margarine until they have reached a softened state, taking around 6 to 7 minutes. Incorporate the mushrooms into the beans, followed by the addition of salt and pepper. Top with ¼ cup bundled seared onions.

8. To prepare green beans, one must properly trim or handle the ends of each individual bean. You can accomplish this by neatly arranging a small handful of beans on the cutting board, followed by skillfully employing a sharp knife to simultaneously remove all the ends.

What Can You Eat?

When it comes to conforming to a dietary regimen, many individuals face a common dilemma - how do we commence our journey? While most individuals possess the ability to discern what to consume, the primary challenge lies in their inability to summon the necessary determination to acquire said items.

begun. If you aspire to embark on a pegan diet, you can commence by adhering to these simple guidelines:.

1. Does the food have natural origins or was it produced by human intervention?

Regardless of the dietary regimen one adheres to, it is imperative to adhere to a single guideline: consume authentic sustenance rather than substances resembling food. Genuine food refers to food items that are devoid of any form of labeling, which may also encompass ingredients that are easily identifiable and pronounceable. This consumable differs minimally in its characteristics from cultivation to consumption.

2. Make an effort to avoid consuming foods that contain excessive labeling. It is necessary for you to abstain from consuming foods with labels. If the ingredients utilized in these food items are commonly found in your culinary space, then they are acceptable.

Furthermore, it is imperative that you abstain from consuming foods that bear labels boasting health and wellness benefits. The labeling of "Heart- Healthy" and "All-Natural" is typically exclusive to processed foods that have undergone extensive refinement. On a bag of broccoli or kale, such labels would assuredly not be visible. The purpose of these wellness cases is to deceive individuals. To provide an illustration, the consumption of potato chips that are free from gluten is not conducive to maintaining good health. In fact, it is unnecessary to make a health claim in order to acknowledge that the consumption of whole vegetables and fruits is beneficial for one's overall wellness.

3. Avoid utilizing ingredients that are difficult to pronounce or would not typically be found in a kitchen setting.

There is a plethora of elements such as artificial sweeteners, MSG, dyes, chemicals, and various ingredients that one would not typically stock in their household. Consequently, what justification could one have for procuring food items that consist of these chemical constituents?

You should consistently avoid consuming foods comprising ingredients whose names are unfamiliar to you, let alone pronouncing them. Refrain from consuming genetically modified organisms (GMOs). 4. Frequently patronize the outer perimeters of the grocery store. Experts recommend purchasing items on the outer edges of a grocery store. By undertaking this action, you will come to comprehend that you are purchasing authentic food products. This designated vicinity is where one can invariably procure wholesome provisions, such as fish, eggs, poultry, red meat, fruits, and vegetables.

In numerous instances, one will encounter processed food-like substances within the central aisles. Therefore, it is advisable to consistently monitor the outer sections of the store, as they tend to offer the newest and most nutritious food options. The sole exceptions pertain to oils, seeds, and nuts that are commonly encountered within the aisles.

5. Eat mostly plant-based foods.

Extensive clinical research has substantiated the presence of a diverse range of health-promoting and therapeutic compounds within plant-derived sources of nutrition. When engaging in the culinary process, it is imperative to consistently take into account the allocation of 75% (by volume) of the dinner plate to include plant-derived food items. It is imperative to consistently incorporate vegetables such as kale, peppers, tomatoes, arugula, bok choy, and broccoli into one's diet. If you are at risk of or have been diagnosed with prediabetes or diabetes, it is advisable to avoid consuming starchy vegetables. In addition, you may consume fruits with a low glycemic index, such as kiwi and berries.

6. Utilizing meat as a condiment, rather than a prominent component of the dish. Although the consumption of meat is permitted within a pegan diet, it does not serve as its focal point. All that is necessary to include in your meal is a modest portion of protein, comparable in size to the palm of your hand, which...

encompasses protein derived from both vegetation and animal sources. When it comes to adhering to a pegan dietary regimen, it is essential to consistently seek out sources of fatty fish, eggs or poultry from pasture-raised animals, and meat from animals raised on a grass-fed diet. In addition, you may wish to consider exploring organic and non-genetically modified tempeh or tofu as an alternative option.

The vegetables should serve as the primary focus on your plate, while meat should be treated as an accompanying component. It is recommended that you consume approximately 4-6 ounces of animal protein on a daily basis.

When engaging in conversation regarding sugar within this vicinity, we are specifically referring to cane sugar, rather than beet sugar. The process involves extracting the vitamins and minerals from sugar cane, resulting in molasses, and whatever remains subsequently becomes white sugar. In order to combat your cravings for sugar, it is imperative to regulate insulin function and maintain stable blood glucose levels. If diminishing cravings for sugar is your objective, it is imperative to eliminate both sugars and grains from your dietary intake. You are able to access internet retailers to search for premium chromium supplements, which can be consumed alongside meals to regulate blood glucose levels and mitigate the desire for sugary foods.

7. Eat fat

Undoubtedly, we acknowledge that the presence of fat is crucial for the optimal functioning of the human physique. It constitutes one of the most essential building elements. In general, it is customary for an individual to consist of approximately 15-30% body fat. Contrary to inaccurate information, it is necessary to consume healthy and balanced fats for optimal fertility, cognitive function, cellular health, and skin quality.

Consumption of unhealthy fats such as refined vegetable oils is not conducive to maintaining good health and wellness. Incorporate a consistent intake of 3-5 portions of nutritious fats such as olive oil, seeds, nuts, and avocados. One individual portion of fat comprises either half of an avocado or a tablespoon's worth of olive oil.

8. Include special super-foods

Any type of food that is abundantly rich in nutrients can be classified as superfoods. A variety of super-foods that should be incorporated into your daily diet have been extensively discussed within this composition. These include fatty fish, grass-fed meat, and plant-based foods. 9. Seek out beans, seeds, and nuts that possess minimal amounts of starch.

Seeds and nuts are commonly found in a typical vegan dietary regimen. Beans are likewise excellent sources of minerals, protein, and dietary fiber; nonetheless, they can also give rise to certain gastrointestinal complications. Individuals with diabetes may encounter significant complications related to their blood glucose levels if they consume a predominantly bean-based diet. One might consider temporarily excluding beans from their diet if they possess an autoimmune disease and/or insulin resistance, as this course of action could prove advantageous.

It is recommended that you adhere to the consumption of low-starch legumes such as lentils, lupine beans, and black beans. Seeds and nuts are highly regarded as popular superfoods.

Incorporating seeds and nuts such as hemp seeds, macadamia nuts, chia seeds, and almonds into your daily dietary regimen would be advisable.

10. Refrain from consuming a large portion of dairy products

The vast majority of paleo and vegan diets do not advocate for the consumption of dairy products. It is recognized to induce various complications such as osteoporosis, cardiovascular ailments, diabetes mellitus, congestion, excessive body weight, and even acne. If one has a preference for dairy products, it is advisable to opt for nutritionally concentrated options such as cheese, goat/sheep yogurt, clarified butter and, additionally, butter.

11. Consistently choose whole grains

Undoubtedly, we do not advocate for the utilization of grains as sustenance; nevertheless, this should not be misconstrued as their detriment to our well-being. When consumed in the form of flours, particularly refined flour, it has the potential to elevate blood glucose levels. It is advised to refrain from consuming gluten derived from flour-based products, as well as daily consumption of heirloom gluten grains such as heirloom rye, einkorn wheat, or barley. However, it should be noted that these heirloom gluten grains are tolerable as long as one does not have gluten sensitivities. However, experts recommend conducting a three-week trial in which you adhere strictly to a gluten-free diet. Subsequently, you may consider reintroducing gluten in order to assess its effects on your well-being. Upon gaining an understanding of the vast improvements associated with adhering to a gluten-free diet, one will undoubtedly develop a profound appreciation for its benefits. There exist specific exceptions, such as the inclusion of nut flour. It is imperative that you abstain from the consumption of flours derived from grains. Consistently incorporate small portions of low-glycemic grains such as quinoa and black rice into your diet. If you are experiencing an autoimmune condition, abdominal adiposity, insulin resistance, or are classified as pre-diabetic/diabetic, it is recommended to completely eliminate grains from your diet for a duration of three weeks and assess the resulting impact on your overall well-being. 12. Indulge in pleasurable culinary delights, albeit not on a daily basis.

A pegan diet plan does not revolve around achieving perfection – over time, it is possible for us to deviate from this daily routine and indulge in some delectable restaurant meals or processed foods. The main objective here is to prevent these minor indulgences from evolving into established habits. You may also savor the occasional indulgence of sugar.

Instead, opt for these indulgences on an occasional basis while adhering to your pegan dietary regimen 90% of the time. If you have a desire for French fries, you can prepare them through the utilization of salt and truffle oil; consequently, you will have the ability to indulge in delectable and uncomplicated French fries. You may indulge in a blended beverage or a glass of red wine in the company of your friends at regular intervals, typically every few weeks or months. It is imperative that you ensure that the occasional indulgences you partake in consist of genuine and whole foods, as opposed to food alternatives that have been previously discussed.

Based on the aforementioned information, it is evident that adhering to a pegan diet can effectively contribute to the restoration of one's personal well-being, as well as the betterment of the overall global health. A pegan diet revolves around a set of uncomplicated principles, each tailored to suit your daily requirements. Incorporating Prominent Superfoods in Your Dietary Regimen The notion of food possessing medicinal properties stands as one of the most potent tools or principles at your disposal for cultivating optimal well-being. Additionally, employing food as a form of medication should be considered as the primary course of action in order to address various types of chronic health conditions. Although there is an extensive array of superfoods accessible in today's market, they can all be classified into distinct categories. Within this domain, we shall undoubtedly explore specific classifications of nourishing foods that are widely regarded as superfoods:

1. Seeds

You must consider three primary types of seeds, namely hemp, chia, and flax. Chia seeds are commonly acknowledged as

An excellent source of omega-3 fatty acids, as well as boasting significantly higher levels of calcium compared to milk. They are likewise an

They are a remarkable reservoir of anti-inflammatory compounds that render them ideal for promoting radiant skin, bolstering mental well-being, and much more.

A single ounce of chia seeds contains roughly 10 grams of fiber. Moreover, the fiber found in chia seeds is insoluble and nourishes beneficial bacteria in the gut, promoting digestive health. Additionally, this fiber undergoes fermentation and produces short-chain fatty acids, which play a crucial role in maintaining gut well-being. Chia seeds not only serve as outstanding sources of healthy proteins, but also possess a higher protein content compared to the majority of plants.

Hemp seeds serve as an exemplary supplementary source of dietary fat and are additionally rich in key nutrients like Vitamin B, protein, magnesium, zinc, and iron. Flax seeds also serve as excellent sources of omega-3 fatty acids, dietary fiber, essential vitamins, and minerals. They also possess potent hormone-balancing substances known as lignans, which exhibit strong anti-cancer properties. Professionals advise incorporating ground flax seeds into your smoothie blends to promote

are facing challenges akin to

irregularity. healthy defecation.

2. MCT oil

MCT oil, derived from coconut oil, is a type of fatty acid commonly referred to as medium-chain triglycerides. Due to its capacity to stimulate lipid metabolism and enhance cognitive function, MCT oil can be regarded as a highly efficacious cellular energy source. As a result of its rapid shedding and metabolism, MCT oil also facilitates weight loss. The oil is readily absorbed directly from the digestive system into the liver, without being stored as adipose tissue, and efficiently converted into energy. MCT oil can be incorporated into various consumable items such as shakes, coffee, salad dressings, and more.

3. Glucomannan

Based on the aforementioned information, it is presently acknowledged that incorporating fiber into your dietary regimen is essential for maintaining optimal health and equilibrium, as well as supplying nourishment to the beneficial microorganisms residing in your gastrointestinal system. In previous times, when humans engaged in both gathering and hunting activities, their average fiber intake amounted to approximately 150 grams, which is significantly higher compared to the relatively low 20 grams consumed at present. Fiber is acknowledged for its ability to mitigate weight issues and other chronic ailments commonly associated with the aging process. This phenomenon occurs as a result of the fiber's ability to regulate the rate of food absorption into the bloodstream, while simultaneously enhancing the speed at which the food passes through the digestive system. Dietary fiber helps maintain optimal levels of blood glucose and cholesterol, facilitates the elimination of toxins from the body, and acts as an appetite suppressant.

It originates from the essence of the cognac, more precisely known as the elephant yam. The cognac tuber has been utilized for countless years as an organic remedy to produce traditional culinary dishes such as brandy-infused noodle delicacies and even the creation of tofu.

A highly effective approach to consume glucomannan is through the utilization of a supplement commonly referred to as PGX. Extensive research has been conducted encompassing diverse subjects such as lipid metabolism, diabetes-related ailments, and implications of cholesterol. "PGX can be incorporated into one's daily water intake, serving as a convenient and dependable source of"

fiber.

4. Mushrooms

It is not merely a singular kind of mushroom; rather, it pertains to the subject matter of mushrooms in our conversation.

the complete range of food items. It is fascinating to observe that an average Chinese individual possesses a greater understanding of the medical properties of various foods compared to many researchers and scientists in the Western hemisphere. This is due to the fact that medical foods are encompassed within their regular dietary consumption.

One of the fundamental components of a Chinese dietary regimen comprises mushrooms such as cordyceps, maitake, shitake, reishi, and others. Each of these various types of mushrooms possess efficacious healing properties, which have the potential to enhance one's immunity and provide sustenance to their hormonal system.

In addition, they possess antiviral and anti-inflammatory properties, and

furthermore, facilitate the restoration of your liver. In addition, mushrooms have the capacity to reduce your cholesterol levels. One could prepare reishi tea or incorporate shitake mushrooms into culinary dishes, particularly in soups.

5. Plant foods

Indeed, the extensive spectrum of hues found in vegetables represents approximately 25,000 compounds and substances that are immensely beneficial for the human body.

- They are commonly referred to as phytochemicals. - The term used to describe them is phytochemicals. - They go by the name phytochemicals. - They are known as phytochemicals in scientific language. - The formal term for them is phytochemicals. There is empirical evidence indicating that the synergistic effects between colors impart supplementary advantages. Consequently, it is recommended that one incorporates a diverse range of colors in their diet, hence the suggestion to "consume the rainbow." It is important to maintain a diversified dietary intake, including a substantial amount of fruits and vegetables with a wide range of colors.

Both vegetables and fruits hold significant importance, both naturally and throughout history. Throughout antiquity, our forebears, the individuals who subsisted through hunting and gathering, ingested an extensive array of over 800 varietals of botanical sustenance. In the present era, our consumption does not come close to that amount.

We should exert further endeavours to incorporate a greater diversity into our daily dietary choices.

Professional opinions consistently affirm the necessity of consuming a diverse range of colorful foods. This can be attributed to the fact that each hue of fruits and vegetables represents distinct groups of therapeutic compounds. Red vegetables, along with fruits such as tomatoes, comprise the carotenoid lycopene, which aids in the elimination of

Free radicals, known to cause genetic damage and inhibit the development of certain types of cancers such as prostate cancer.

cancer.

Conversely, vegetables and fruits that are environmentally sustainable contain compounds such as isocyanates, indels, and Fleur Fane, all of which contribute to cancer prevention through the inhibition and elimination of carcinogens within the body.

Based on the aforementioned, it is imperative to endeavor each and every one of them, including purple, yellow, orange, white, blue, and other such hues. All of these vegetables and fruits possess remarkable benefits.

In order to restrict access to this portion, it is recommended by experts that you adhere to a daily regimen of medication consumption. Incorporating these types of nutrient-dense foods into one's diet is consistently a significantly superior choice. Please consider that these foods have inherent properties that surpass those of any substances typically found in prescription medications.

Precautions To Take On The Pagan Diet

After elucidating and analyzing the fundamental constitution of the Pegan diet, there are additional considerations regarding the items to abstain from for individuals embarking on the Pegan diet. These guidelines hold significant importance, particularly for beginners. It is crucial to duly acknowledge and take into consideration the aspects that must be avoided.

In adherence to the principles of the Pegan diet, it is recommended to decrease the overall consumption of grains. Whole grains that have undergone processing should be steered clear of, particularly by individuals aiming to adhere strictly to the dietary guidelines of the Pegan diet. Nonetheless, for newcomers seeking to fully integrate into this meal plan, it is advisable to opt for organic, freshly produced grains, while ensuring a substantial inclusion of vegetables in the mix. Consuming gluten-free grains in moderation can contribute to improved digestive health. It is advisable to consume organic vegetables alongside grains such as millet, quinoa, and teff. Indeed, solely whole grains that are devoid of gluten are deemed permissible. They may manifest as wheat bread, biscuits, or a millet-based beverage.

Furthermore, it is important to gradually transition the focal point of your meals towards consuming clean, natural, and unprocessed food. It is advisable to primarily consume foods that are minimally processed or resemble their natural state. Prior to consuming, it would be prudent to inquire within oneself or ascertain the degree of authenticity in which a desired protein, vegetable, or nutritious fat retains its inherent state. Opt for locally sourced and organic food in 90% of instances.

Following the Pegan diet may not pose considerable difficulty, and its benefits may manifest earlier than anticipated when refraining from the consumption of chemicals, additives, preservatives, all processed food, and notably, sugar. Indeed, the consumption of sugar should be limited to occasional indulgences or what is commonly known as a "cheat day." Moreover, it is advisable to refrain from the regular consumption of various pasta dishes, as well as highly processed and excessively seasoned snacks. Nevertheless, for novice individuals, should they choose to prepare pasta, it is advisable that the pasta portion constitute only approximately one-eighth of the overall plate, with the remaining portion comprising an assortment of various vegetables. Subsequently, it is recommended that your subsequent meals following the pasta dish comprise of an assortment of vegetables, legumes, and predominantly plant-based fare. If you have a desire for a snack, you can opt for a fruit salad incorporating vegetables, accompanied by nuts such as granola, tiger nuts, dates, and a modest selection of berries.

Significantly, it is crucial to note that while the Pegan diet incorporates a combination of plant-based foods and animal-derived proteins, it is equally important to abstain from the consumption of dairy products. The consumption of dairy products derived from cows and other animals should be minimized as much as possible. In lieu of this, consider selecting dairy alternatives derived from plants, such as coconut milk, tiger nut drink, almond milk, and other plant-based options sourced from nuts and seeds.

Incorporating unprocessed sweet potatoes into your Pegan dietary regimen is advisable for a well-rounded meal plan. Additionally, the fats consumed should incorporate sources abundant in Omega 3 such as oily fish and oil derived from nuts. Moreover, coconut oils serve as a remarkable option for facilitating healthy fat intake, being a notable reservoir of saturated fat that is quintessential for incorporating into the Pegan diet. It is advisable to refrain from consuming starchy legumes such as peanuts. Nevertheless, lentils can be incorporated into your dietary regimen.

One should abstain from the consumption of refined oils and ultra-processed meals, including canola oil, soybean oil, sunflower oil, and corn oils when adhering to the Pegan diet meal plan. Once you have made the commitment to adhere to the Pegan diet, it is advised to abstain from consuming artificial colorings in food and desserts, along with other chemical preservatives.

The foods that are recommended to be avoided in the Pegan diet primarily stem from their detrimental effects on blood sugar levels, which, upon elevation, can potentially contribute to the development of conditions such as diabetes or provoke inflammation within the body.

"Morning Meal Ideas Suitable for the Pegan Dietary Approach:

01. Smoothie containing strawberries, bananas, and coconut milk.

This smoothie offers a delectable flavor combination of strawberries and cream. The texture of this dish is exceptionally velvety due to the inclusion of coconut milk. Furthermore, strawberries bestow upon dishes a conventional flavor profile and a gentle blush of pale pink color. The sweetness in this coconut milk smoothie is derived solely from a frozen ripe banana, without the addition of any additional sweeteners.

A helpful suggestion: freeze overly ripe bananas to have them readily available for blending into smoothies. It is common practice to remove the peels from bananas prior to freezing, allowing them to be stored as whole fruits or sliced into smaller pieces. Bananas that have undergone the process of freezing can be easily sliced or divided into chunks as desired.

Certainly, should you desire a strawberry smoothie with fewer carbohydrates, it is possible to exclude the banana and add sweeteners such as stevia, monk fruit, or any other sweetener that is low in carbohydrates, to your preferred level of sweetness. In this particular situation, I would opt for frozen strawberries along with a couple of ice cubes to maintain the low temperature of the smoothie. Furthermore, I would include coconut cream, extracted from the upper layer of a refrigerated can of coconut milk, to enhance its smooth and creamy texture.

In order to attain the exceptionally thick texture, it is recommended to utilize coconut milk with a high fat content. Please contemplate acquiring coconut milk that is stored in a container devoid of contaminants such as a BPA-free can or carton. The roster of constituents should exclusively comprise of coconut and water. It is advisable to refrain from consuming refrigerated coconut milk due to its common inclusion of gums or other refined food additives, as it poses a greater safety risk.

The inclusion of vanilla extract bestows a taste reminiscent of an ice cream confection upon this recipe for strawberry banana smoothie, evoking the nostalgia of a classic strawberry milkshake. I employ organic vanilla paste in my preparations, although alternative options include vanilla powder or the extraction of seeds from a vanilla bean.

02. Eggs and Zoodles Cooked in the Oven Served with Avocado as a Nutrient-Dense Meal in Alignment with a Ketogenic Dietary Regimen

With an abundance of meat and cheese at one's disposal, the keto diet is undeniably rich in savory flavors. Nonetheless, there are instances when one desires something that does not bestow an equally burdensome feeling. Introducing ketogenic style fried eggs served with avocado zoodles. They possess a notable amount of fats and proteins and serve as an optimal choice to enhance morning or evening meals.

Instructions:

1. Kindly ensure that the oven is preheated to a temperature of 350 degrees Fahrenheit. Apply a thin layer of nonstick oil to a baking sheet.

2. Combine the zucchini noodles and olive oil in a large bowl, ensuring they are thoroughly mixed. Enhance the flavor with a sprinkle of sea salt and a dash of freshly ground pepper. Partition the amalgamation into four equivalent portions, transfer them onto the arranged baking sheet, and mold each portion into a nest-like shape.

3. Delicately break an egg into the foundation of each individual nest. Proceed with baking for a duration of 9 to 11 minutes, or until the eggs have attained the desired level of readiness. Season with salt and pepper according to personal preference; adorn with a sprinkling of red pepper flakes and basil as a final touch. Accompany of avocado slices.

03. Vegan Vegetable Frittata

The Vegan Frittata is a superb means of utilizing surplus vegetables and crafting an uncomplicated, cost-effective vegan dish that is befitting for any mealtime, including breakfast, lunch, or even dinner!

Frittata is a customary Italian culinary creation comprising of eggs and various seasonal vegetables. In this vegan variation, we will utilize a highly flavorful tofu-based "egg" mixture and ample amounts of vegetables to craft a truly delightful vegan frittata.

Ingredients Needed

In this recipe, a blend of tofu and spices are smoothly pureed to produce a 'egg' preparation, which is subsequently combined with sautéed vegetables. The concoction is subsequently subjected to baking until a golden crust forms on the exterior, while the interior retains a tender consistency, culminating in an exquisite vegetarian vegan frittata.

Herein is a comprehensive list of all the items that will be necessary, accompanied by recommendations for potential ingredient replacements:

Potatoes of varying hues, such as white, red, gold, and russet (with or without the peel), are all suitable options.

Any onion of any color would be suitable.

Utilize bell peppers with your preferred taste for this recipe.

Cauliflower florets "

Replace the yellow squash with a few halved cherry tomatoes.

Garlic (Allium sativum) is a pungent bulbous plant belonging to the Allium genus and is widely cultivated for both culinary and medicinal purposes.

Silken tofu, both solid and soft varieties, preferably organic. All types of tofu exhibit a slightly gritty texture when blended, requiring personal exploration to discover a variety that satisfies your palate. In most cases, silken tofu does not exhibit a chalky taste. There is no necessity to exert pressure on the tofu ingredient.

Unsweetened plant-based milk can be used as a substitute for dairy milk according to your preference.

Cornstarch, preferably of organic origin, may be replaced with arrowroot or tapioca flour.

Nutritional yeast

Mustard options include dijon or whole grain mustard (or substitute with mustard powder).

Tarragon can be replaced with thyme, basil, or a combination of the two.

Garlic in powdered form

The spice known as turmeric

Red pepper flakes.

Add a sprinkle of salt and pepper for seasoning.

Vegan Frittata Preparation

01. Ensure that the oven is preheated to a temperature of 375 degrees Fahrenheit.

02. To commence, prepare the tofu egg mixture by amalgamating the tofu, nutritional yeast, dijon, cornstarch, garlic powder, herbs, red pepper flakes, and salt and pepper in the bowl of a food

processor or blender and blending until velvety, while intermittently scraping down the sides.

03. Next, proceed to cook the vegetables on the stovetop.

04. After the ingredients are properly prepared, integrate the sauce mixture with the cooked vegetables.

05. Ultimately, pour the vegan vegetable frittata mixture into a 9-inch springform pan, filling it halfway. Alternatively, any shallow dish measuring 9 x 11 will suffice.

06. Please proceed to bake for approximately 40 to 45 minutes. The frittata displayed in the image was prepared for the full duration of 45 minutes.

07. And just like magic, you now have a scrumptious vegan frittata ready to be served to your loved ones.

04. Asparagus and Tomato Egg Dish

Kindly indicate by means of raising your hand if you have a fondness for eggs. Now, should you have a disdain for sweeping, please raise the alternative. With that purpose in mind, may I present to you a culinary creation that is poised to become your ultimate preferred recipe. This sheet-pan egg dish represents an optimal choice for both breakfast and dinner.

How to Prepare:

1. Please ensure that the oven is heated to a temperature of 400 degrees Fahrenheit in advance. Apply nonstick cooking oil to the baking dish.
2. Systematically distribute the asparagus and cherry tomatoes across the baking sheet, ensuring an uniform arrangement. Add a sprinkle of thyme and a pinch of salt and pepper according to personal preference. Pour the olive oil evenly onto the vegetables.
3. Roast the asparagus and tomatoes for a duration of 10 to 12 minutes, or until the asparagus reaches a state of partial tenderness and the tomatoes display a wrinkled appearance.

4. Ensure that each egg is properly seasoned with a sprinkle of salt and pepper atop the asparagus.

5. Proceed to place the dish back into the oven and continue baking for an additional 7 to 8 minutes, or until the egg whites have set while leaving the yolks with a slight jiggle.

6. Allocate an equal portion of asparagus, onions, and eggs into individual plates, ensuring there are four servings.

Is It Feasible To Adhere To The Pegan Diet While Pregnant?

In the upcoming chapter, we shall address a specific requirement pertaining to the Pegan diet, namely the dietary needs of expectant mothers. Prior to presenting these recommendations, it is essential to consider whether this particular dietary regimen is suitable for expectant mothers.

Affirmative, albeit with certain reservations.

What does it mean? It signifies that this dietary regimen is compatible with the aforementioned timeframe, albeit necessitating certain precautions.

Consequently, pregnant women will need to make dietary adjustments in accordance with the specific requirements and necessities of this particular phase.

Indeed, there is a widespread recommendation to refrain from adopting a weight-reduction diet while pregnant or during the period of breastfeeding. There remains a prevalent belief among many individuals that one must consume food for two people during pregnancy. Nevertheless, this assertion is entirely false. Throughout the duration of pregnancy, it is possible to adhere to a nutritious and well-rounded dietary regimen, whilst ensuring one's satiety needs are adequately met. It is crucial to adhere to certain fundamental guidelines and precautionary measures. Due to this rationale, we have allocated a section exclusively tailored to accommodate the implementation of this dietary regimen during this exceptionally sensitive period of a woman's life.

Valuable advice and strategies for expectant mothers

After providing a brief preamble on the appropriateness of adhering to this dietary regimen while pregnant, let us now proceed to furnish you with some pragmatic guidance should you find it necessary to embrace this diet for the betterment of your well-being and that of your unborn child.

If you intend to adhere to this dietary regimen throughout your pregnancy, there are undoubtedly numerous concerns and uncertainties that arise. The aforementioned reservations or doubts stem directly from the overarching dietary guidelines pertaining to pregnancy.

If you desire to adhere to this dietary plan, it is imperative to reduce, if not entirely eradicate, certain components or ingredients.

• Firstly, the consumption of raw protein foods should be avoided entirely, as this rule applies universally to all pregnant individuals. However, in the case of this dietary regimen which incorporates animal-derived proteins, it is crucial that your foods are prepared thoroughly and cooked to perfection. Consequently, tartare, carpaccio, and raw sausages are not available. Consuming uncooked fish is strictly prohibited. Animal proteins in their raw state are strictly avoided due to the potential transmission of pathogenic bacteria such as Salmonella or Listeria Monocytogenes, as well as parasites like Toxoplasma Gondii. These microorganisms are known to cause foodborne infections or adverse health conditions in developing embryos. Hence, it is imperative to steer clear of specific foods and cooking techniques while pregnant, and diligently adhere to established principles of food safety. The same goes for eggs even if in this diet, as we will see in the following chapters, only eggs of biological origin are consumed. Despite their origin, it is imperative that they are never consumed in their raw state. In addition, when it comes to milk, it is advisable to always subject it to a process of boiling.

• It is advised to refrain from consuming smoked foods, particularly products of animal origin. Limiting or completely eliminating the consumption of smoked sausages or smoked fish is highly recommended.

In terms of fish, it is advisable to make a concerted effort to diminish the intake of large predatory fish and limit tuna consumption to no more than twice per week, specifically during pregnancy. This is essential to minimize the potential exposure to heavy metals like mercury, as well as pollutants. Alternatively, it is advisable to opt for fish varieties such as sole, cod, hake, trout, red snapper, and sea bream.

• In regards to vegetables and fruit, which are foundational components of the Vegan diet, it is essential to address the potential issue of inadequate cleanliness during pregnancy. Consequently, it becomes imperative to thoroughly cleanse each vegetable prior to consumption. Furthermore, it is imperative to exclude the vegetables packaged in bags. It will be necessary to select solely fresh produce that can be thoroughly washed and inspected. The consumption of uncooked vegetables should be restricted as a precautionary measure against potential bacterial contamination and associated illnesses. Hence, it is always advisable to employ diligent care in thoroughly cleansing fruits and vegetables prior to ingestion, cutting, or culinary preparations (even those intended for peeling). This can be achieved by employing a stream of tap water or, for optimal efficacy, chlorine-based cleansing agents (bearing in mind that bicarbonate is not effetive). When employing chlorine-based detergents, it is advisable to not restrict the cleaning process to mere immersion in a solution of water and detergent, but rather to rinse the produce under a steady flow of running water.

A general principle applicable to both Pegan and pregnancy is the unequivocal prohibition on the consumption of alcohol, which poses a risk to the well-being of the developing fetus. Moreover, when it comes to Pegan, it is necessary to restrict the intake of tea and coffee as well. If you find it absolutely necessary, limit your intake to a maximum of one cup, but ensure that they are exclusively decaffeinated.

The aforementioned are all the constraints to adhere to in a universal sense during pregnancy, with particular emphasis placed on their significance should one choose to embrace the principles of the Pegan diet.

Regarding all the additional information that should be included, we aim to provide you with a brief overview.

Firstly, as previously delineated, it is imperative to dispel the notion that during pregnancy one should consume double the amount of food. Quite the opposite, the overall daily caloric intake should be only marginally increased, alongside the maintenance of weight control. However, it is essential to augment the intake of certain nutrients, particularly vitamins and minerals. To effectively manage the escalating nutritional demands, adhering to a diversified dietary regimen, comprising fresh and seasonal produce, partitioned into 4 or 5 servings throughout the day, is crucial. This approach ensures an abundant supply of essential vitamins and minerals. Additionally, it is advisable to meet a daily hydration goal of consuming a minimum of two liters of water. Due to this rationale, it is imperative that we, subsequent to establishing this premise, supplement our discussion pertaining to the Pegan diet during pregnancy. Prior to providing these suggestions, it is imperative for us to offer a fundamental piece of advice: irrespective of the specific dietary approach you may choose, it is vital to seek the expert opinion of a medical professional when considering the adoption of the Pegan diet. Never overlook this detail.

After establishing this point and setting forth this premise, it is essential to outline the necessary adjustments one must make to adhere to the Pegan lifestyle during pregnancy.

• Bear in mind the appropriate quantity of carbohydrates: if you intend to adhere to this dietary regimen, it is necessary to incorporate carbohydrates into your meals. Give preference to whole grains derived from organic sources and legumes. Certainly, should you wish to adhere to a specific dietary regimen, it is imperative to avoid overindulging in the converse direction. The focus consistently lies on maintaining equilibrium between serving sizes and macronutrient composition.

• Incorporate a greater amount of lean proteins into your diet: it is advisable to prioritize lean meats and white fish as protein sources.

• It is imperative to enhance the intake of cooked vegetables: as previously mentioned, one must increase their vegetable consumption, ensuring that they are thoroughly washed and properly cooked.

• One may adhere to this dietary plan despite occasional lapses: it is permissible to indulge in homemade desserts occasionally, provided they strictly adhere to the principles of Pegan, wherein all ingredients must be organic and verified.

• Ensure that you incorporate vitamins and minerals into your diet if they are necessary for your overall well-being. In the context of a dietary regimen, it is widely acknowledged that nutritional deficiencies can potentially occur. The vegan diet has been meticulously formulated to address the deficiencies in vitamins, minerals, and fiber typically found in more drastic dietary approaches. Nevertheless, whilst pregnant, the substantial consumption of vegetables and proteins might prove insufficient. Furthermore, in accordance with medical guidance, it is recommended to incorporate folic acid, as well as vitamins and iron supplements, into your dietary regimen.

These are all the necessary measures that should be taken into consideration in order to modify this diet to suit pregnancy. The upcoming chapter will include an exclusive segment focused entirely on the Pegan diet, the amalgamation of sports and how they intertwine.

Some Pegan Diet Rules

As previously indicated, the Pegan diet draws inspiration from two prominent dietary approaches - the paleo and vegan diets. "Per Dr. Hyman's analysis, this dietary plan endeavors to enhance overall well-being by harmonizing the blood sugar levels and

lessening irritation. To grasp the principles of adhering to a Pegan diet, they encompass:

1. Select vegetables and fruits that are in season.

The primary dietary requirement for adhering to a Pegan diet is comprised of leafy foods, which should constitute approximately 75% of your plate. To be honest, it is imperative that they constitute a considerable portion of your daily dietary intake. They encompass essential minerals and nutrients that promote physical well-being and provide protection against ailments.

The adoption of a diet rich in vegetables and organic products stands to benefit the majority of individuals, promoting a vibrant, healthy, and well-balanced lifestyle. Vegetables and organic products encompass a diverse array of minerals and nutrients that greatly promote one's well-being, including folic acid, phosphorus, zinc, magnesium, as well as various vitamins such as E, C, A (beta-carotene), and others.

Fruits and vegetables also exhibit low sugar, salt, and fat content. They serve as considerable sources of dietary fibers and possess a low caloric content. By incorporating fruits and vegetables into your diet, you will be able to maintain a healthy weight and reduce obesity. In addition, you will also reduce your blood pressure and cholesterol levels.

Fruits and vegetables are abundant in potent phytochemicals that contribute to the maintenance of your overall well-being. Phytochemicals are primarily associated with pigmentation - hence, it can be inferred that vegetables and fruits displaying a range of colors such as white, blue-purple, red, yellow-orange, and green possess distinct combinations of nutrients and phytochemicals that synergistically contribute to the promotion of overall well-being. For instance, it is worth noting that white vegetables such as cauliflower possess sulforaphane, which potentially contributes to the protection against certain forms of tumors. Conversely, green vegetables like kale and spinach contain zeaxanthin and lutein, both of which offer protection against age-related ailments such as eye diseases. We will delve further into the topic of the Rainbow diet in subsequent sections.

If it is essential to enhance dietary intake, it is vital to incorporate a diverse range of fruits and vegetables. One could consider seeking out fruits and vegetables based on seasonal availability, as this ensures a balanced intake of nutrients and natural compounds provided by nature.

Alternatively, you may also choose to purchase a variety of fruits and vegetables and experiment with new culinary creations.

2. Quality is Important

The food items that are notable within the context of a Pegan diet can be considered as authentic sources of nourishment - these culinary options are abundant in nutrients, devoid of chemical additives, and predominantly organic in nature. Typically, these are the types of dietary sources that were commonly consumed by ancient civilizations. Regrettably, processed food options surged in popularity during the twentieth century and underwent a substantial shift towards pre-packaged, ready-to-consume meals.

Although convenient and efficient, processed food options can also be detrimental to one's well-being. Undoubtedly, consuming authentic sources of high quality nutrition can be one of the foremost actions one can take for the betterment of their physical well-being, thereby ensuring a superior quality of life. The composition of the food varieties you consume will significantly impact your overall health.

In the context of any dietary regimen, the quality of the foods and ingredients is of paramount importance. Fundamentally, the character of the food sources adhered to in a Pegan diet ought to consist solely of remarkable options. A typical Pegan dish necessitates the inclusion of 2-3 fresh portions of produce, consisting of leafy greens, dark-colored vegetables, and other non-monotonous varieties. In order to achieve optimal nutritional density, it is advised to incorporate a variety of vibrant vegetables and fruits into your diet. Due to the adoption of a Pegan diet, emphasis on food quality is a crucial nutritional factor. Therefore, it is advisable to consistently opt for organic and locally sourced food options whenever available.

Moreover, the Pegan diet incorporates several animal-derived components. In any event, these culinary preparations are meant to be employed as complementary accompaniments to the plant-based main courses. The eggs, poultry, and red meat should be produced using humane and sustainable farming practices, such as organic or pasture-raised methods. It is recommended that the fish be captured from their natural habitat, as this would result in reduced levels of mercury contamination.

Omega-3 unsaturated fats are also included as a component of the Pegan diet, given their highly recognized anti-inflammatory properties. These types of cuisine typically feature fish, preferably selected from the plentiful range of wild-caught oily fishes such as herring, mackerel, anchovies, sardines, and salmon.

3. Plant-based Foods Should Constitute 75% of Your Overall Food Intake

Consumption

The Pegan diet combines the principles of both a paleo diet and a vegetarian diet. The paleolithic diet consists of whole foods that our ancestors hunted and gathered, such as vegetables, fruits, nuts, and occasionally meat. On the other hand, the vegetarian diet entails consuming solely plant-based foods.

According to the guidelines, a Pegan diet is defined as a dietary pattern in which 75% of the food consumed consists of plant-based sources, while the remaining 25% is derived from animal-based proteins. These food sources are required to be fully and efficiently produced, while minimizing their impact on the environment.

While comprehensive investigations providing evidence of the advantages of a Pegan diet remain inconclusive, experts are accumulating data that indicates the favorable impact of this semi-plant-based dietary approach on one's health. Given that a plant-based diet prioritizes the consumption of vegetables and fruits that are low in carbohydrates and rich in dietary fiber, the Pegan diet is widely regarded as the most optimal dietary approach in contemporary times. Research has also focused on the notion that a diet predominantly based on plants can effectively reduce levels of unhealthy cholesterol in the body and facilitate the process of weight reduction.

Vegetables and organic produce are widely recognized as the most nutritionally diverse food categories available today, as they boast the highest concentration of minerals and nutrients. Consumption of these foods is known to play a crucial role in disease prevention, as well as the reduction of both inflammation and oxidative stress.

However, it is pertinent to avoid certain types of plant-based food sources. For instance, white bread and rice also fall under the category of plant-based food options. Nevertheless, they are handled in a profound manner which indicates the absence of essential nutrients and a high glycemic index. Therefore, this can lead to heightened appetite (resulting in overeating) and elevated blood sugar levels.

An additional 25% of the dietary intake is made up of proteins derived from animal sources. However, it is advisable to keep the portion sizes small, treating all the meat dishes as accompanying sides. The meat should be sourced from animals that were raised in pasture-based systems and fed a natural grass diet. Regarding fish, it is imperative that they originate from natural habitats and exhibit minimal levels of mercury.

4. Eat the Rainbow

For optimal nutritional intake, experts recommend incorporating a wide variety of colorful fruits and vegetables into your diet. As previously indicated, this implies that one should consume vibrant vegetables and fruits that are organic in nature. Such attributes offer numerous benefits for one's physical well-being.

Flora encompasses a manifold of hues, commonly referred to as phytonutrients. These phytonutrients afford them a broad range of hues. Various types of fruits and vegetables have frequently been associated with specific health benefits and nutritional value. Although consuming ample quantities of leafy greens is highly beneficial, it is equally imperative to emphasize the consumption of diverse botanicals, rich in various nutrients that support overall well-being.

Although phytonutrients offer numerous benefits, conducting randomized controlled trials can be challenging. As a result, researchers have relied on observational studies to analyze the association between phytonutrient intake and the risk of developing diseases within a population. Based on the findings of these examinations, it has been observed that consuming vibrant vegetables and natural products offers numerous benefits, with minimal drawbacks. By incorporating a range of shades into your Pegan diet, you will provide your body with a diverse array of phytochemicals, minerals, and vitamins.

Allow us to explore several tones and examine their potential health advantages: Starting with the color red.

Fruits and vegetables encompass grapefruit, pink guava, watermelon, tomato, and so forth.

Primary phytonutrient: Lycopene (belonging to the Vitamin A family)

Additionally, there are other essential minerals and vitamins:

Vitamin K1

Vitamin C

Potassium

Folate

Health benefits:

Reduces the likelihood of specific forms of cancer

Reduce sun-related skin damage

Improves heart health

Yellow and orange

Fruits and vegetables encompass a variety of winter squash, pumpkin, bananas, tangerines, pineapple, carrots, yellow peppers, and more.

Primary phytonutrient: Carotenoids (belonging to the Vitamin A family)

Additional minerals and vitamins:

Vitamin C

Potassium

Vitamin A

Folate

Fiber

Health benefits:

Reduces the likelihood of developing cancer

Supports

Eye health

Improves heart health

Green

Fruits and vegetables encompass a variety of verdant herbs and produce, such as Brussel sprouts, green cabbage, asparagus, avocados, broccoli, kale, spinach, and more.

Primary plant compounds: Carotenoids and chlorophyll found in leafy vegetables, and glucosinolates, isothiocyanates, and indoles present in cruciferous vegetables such as cabbage and broccoli.

Additional minerals and vitamins:

Vitamin K1

Vitamin A

Potassium

Magnesium

Folate Fiber

Health benefits:

Reduces the likelihood of developing cardiovascular disorders and malignancies.

Antioxidant

Anti-inflammatory

5. Avoid Gluten

The phrases 'gluten-free' and 'dairy-free' have been emerging ubiquitously.

in the previous few years. Many individuals who are currently not reliant on gluten products have managed to regulate chronic conditions, food intolerances, and

aggravation. Dairy and gluten are typical allergens that can give rise to a multitude of medical complications in individuals.

Gluten can be classified as a specific type of protein known as a prolamin, which is commonly present in various grains such as rye, barley, and wheat. Gluten is commonly referred to as a "remarkable" substance that imparts cohesiveness to processed food items due to its renowned elasticity. There are several mechanisms through which gluten can induce inflammation within the body. The reason for this is that it contains significant amounts of anti-nutrients, specifically proteins present in certain varieties of plants.

These adversaries of supplements are detrimental to the body as they hinder the natural process of food assimilation and absorption in the stomach, thereby resulting in inflammation.

The consumption of gluten also leads to the production of zonulin within the body. Zonulin is a protein present in the body that regulates the opening and closing of the junctions within the gastric mucosa. The stomach exhibits porosity, selectively facilitating the absorption of beneficial substances into the bloodstream while retaining detrimental elements for subsequent elimination. By inhibiting zonulin, the permeability of the stomach will be reduced, thereby preventing closure of the junctions.

Dairy refers to animal milk like sheep's milk, goat's milk, cow's milk, and even camel's milk. Dairy is also present in a broad range of other commodities such as butter, cheese, kefir, yogurt, and cream. Dairy is classified as an allergenic food that poses difficulties in digestion, thereby leading to the occurrence of inflammation.

For example, lactose prejudice is a condition that stems from dairy. Lactose, a type of sugar present in milk, necessitates the production of the enzyme lactase for its metabolism in the body. This protein is synthesized endogenously during the early stages of life, and its production diminishes gradually as we progress through the aging process. This is a highly prevalent condition - over 65% of adults globally display lactose intolerance.

Dairy products also encompass casein, a protein that may contribute to certain implications regarding immune system functionality and digestion, particularly the presence of A1 casein. If you are of the belief that lactose and A1 casein are contributing to digestive discomfort, it would be advisable to explore alternative options within the realm of dairy products. As an illustration, it can be observed that goat's milk possesses a lower lactose content compared to that of cow's milk.

6. Reject the Use of Vegetable Oils "

It is not widely known, yet vegetable oils have detrimental effects on both human health and the environment. Vegetable oils are oils that are derived from various plant sources.

Various types of seeds such as nuts, safflower, sunflower, corn, soybean, and rapeseed (commonly known as canola oil) are included. Unlike olive oil and coconut oil, which are extracted through mechanical pressing, these vegetable oils undergo unnatural extraction methods.

In addition to persisting misconceptions concerning cholesterol and saturated fats, these oils are frequently marketed as being healthful due to their inclusion of omega-3 fatty acids and monounsaturated fats. Progressions will often focus specifically on these fraudulent health assertions. Nevertheless, this does not encapsulate the entire viewpoint.

It is a well-established fact that vegetable oils possess elevated levels of polyunsaturated fats (PUFAs), while the human body is composed of approximately 97%

Monounsaturated and fully saturated fatty acids. Fat is essential for the synthesis of hormones and the regeneration of cells. Conversely, polyunsaturated fatty acids (PUFAs) exhibit a high degree of instability and are prone to rapid oxidation. Consequently, this can lead to cellular mutation and inflammation. The process of oxidation has also been associated with other cardiac-related diseases.

Undoubtedly, it is widely acknowledged that omega-3 fatty acids possess considerable health benefits. Nevertheless, the crucial factor for maintaining optimum health lies in the balance between omega-3 and omega-6 acids.

Vegetable oils are abundant in omega-6 fatty acids. These acids undergo rapid oxidation. Conversely, omega-3 fatty acids have demonstrated a propensity to provide safeguard against cancer and mitigate inflammation. There is a correlation between imbalanced levels of both types of acids and various forms of cancers as well as other health complications.

In addition to the atypical concentrations of omega-6 fatty acids and polyunsaturated fats, these vegetable oils encompass various substances such as chemicals, pesticides, and processing additives. Additionally, certain variants include BHT and BHA as well, which serve as natural antioxidants that effectively inhibit food deterioration. Nevertheless, research has demonstrated that they also generate potentially carcinogenic compounds within the physiological system. In conclusion, vegetable oil is additionally associated with adverse effects such as renal and hepatic impairment, cognitive and behavioral abnormalities, reproductive challenges, and compromised immune function.

7. Refrain from consuming excessive amounts of sugar and ensure a balanced intake of fruits

From peanut butter to marinara sauce, nearly all products contain added sugar. The majority of individuals depend on processed foods for their consumption of snacks and meals. Nevertheless, these products are also comprised of additional sugar, constituting a significant portion of their overall caloric consumption.

Per the recommendations outlined in dietary guidelines, it is advisable to restrict the consumption of added sugar to no more than 10% of your daily calorie intake. The excessive intake of sugar has been deemed a primary factor contributing to the development of obesity, as well as a potential catalyst for various chronic ailments including Type-2 diabetes.

The prevalence of obesity is experiencing an unprecedented rise, with one of the primary contributing factors being the consumption of sugar-sweetened beverages. Beverages containing high amounts of added sugar, such as sweet tea, fruit juice, and carbonated sodas, are known to contain fructose, a type of simple sugar. The ingestion of fructose elicits an augmentation in one's appetite. Moreover, the consumption of fructose contributes to an increased level of resistance towards leptin, a hormone responsible for appetite regulation and signaling satiety to the body.

To summarize succinctly, it can be asserted that sweetened beverages fail to satiate hunger and instead contribute to the intake of excessive calories in liquid form, leading to an undesirable increase in body weight. Studies have established a correlation between the consumption of sugary beverages and higher body weight in individuals.

Consuming excessive quantities of sugar in your diet can also elevate the likelihood of developing cardiovascular conditions. Extensive research has demonstrated that diets rich in sugar have the potential to induce inflammation, contribute to obesity, and elevate blood pressure, all of which constitute risk factors for a range of cardiovascular conditions.

An association has been identified between elevated sugar intake and the occurrence of acne. Foods characterized by a elevated glycemic index, such as processed sugary delicacies, elicit a more rapid elevation of blood sugar levels compared to those foods with a lower glycemic index. Consuming these foods can elicit significant fluctuations in insulin and blood sugar levels, thereby triggering heightened inflammation, increased production of skin oils, and elevated secretion of androgens. These physiological responses are directly implicated in the development of acne. Moreover, extensive investigations on population patterns have revealed that rural communities across the globe, who adhere to a non-processed food diet, exhibit significantly lower occurrences of acne when compared to affluent urban locales.

8. Avoid Gluten Grains

As previously stated, gluten is an inherent protein present in certain grains such as rye, barley, and wheat. This substance possesses an elastic attribute that promotes cohesion of the food components. Other grains that contain gluten include triticale, einkorn, Khorasan wheat, graham, farro, farina, semolina, emmer, durum, spelt, and wheat berries. Although oats are inherently free of gluten, the presence of gluten arises from cross-contamination during their processing alongside the aforementioned cereals. Additional, more subtle sources of gluten encompass modified food starch and soy sauce.

An unfavorable aspect of gluten is its potential to elicit adverse reactions in certain individuals. Individuals may exhibit varied reactions to gluten, as their bodies perceive it as a harmful substance, prompting the activation of the immune system to combat it. In the event that one possesses sensitivity towards gluten and inadvertently ingests it, this will lead to the manifestation of inflammation. The potential adverse effects encompass a spectrum, ranging from mild manifestations such as diarrhea, alternating constipation, bloating, and fatigue, to more severe consequences including intestinal impairment, malnutrition, and unintended weight loss.

An estimation suggests that around 0.9% of the American population is affected by celiac disease. Furthermore, it has been determined that individuals with celiac disease face an increased susceptibility to anemia and osteoporosis. Furthermore, this phenomenon gives rise to an array of additional health complications such as disorders in the nervous system, diminished fertility, and potentially even the development of malignancies.

The favorable information is that the harm can be rectified by the mere omission of gluten from your dietary intake. Selecting a diet that excludes gluten is frequently the resolution for individuals with celiac disease. Nonetheless, adhering to a gluten-free regimen proves to be a formidable undertaking; it may be necessary to seek counsel from a certified nutritionist in order to ascertain both the presence of gluten in various food sources and the proper substitution of essential nutrients through gluten-free alternatives.

In essence, a gluten-free diet entails the exclusion of food items that contain gluten from one's consumption. On the other hand, the majority of gluten-containing whole grains boast essential nutrients such as iron, magnesium, and vitamins. As a result, it is crucial that you compensate for these deficient nutrients. For instance, one may explore naturally gluten-free dietary options such as poultry, eggs, fish, nuts, and whole fruits and vegetables.

9. Include Healthy Fats

The majority of individuals struggle to comprehend the reasons behind the favorable effects of monounsaturated and polyunsaturated fats on the body, as well as the adverse impact of trans fats. Indeed, our objective has been to minimize the consumption of fats in your dietary intake by transitioning towards meals that incorporate reduced levels of fat. Nevertheless, this alteration does not enhance our well-being as it entails a reduction in the consumption of beneficial fats while increasing intake of detrimental fats.

While certain types of fats may have adverse effects on the human body, there are also essential fats that play a vital role. Dietary fats play a crucial role as a primary source of energy for the human organism. It will aid in the assimilation of various minerals and vitamins. Fatty substances also play a role in the formation of protective coverings surrounding the nerves and cellular membranes. Lipids also serve to aid in the processes of inflammation, muscular contractions, and coagulation. Hence, certain types of fats exhibit more desirable effects on the body over an extended period of time.

Irrespective of their quality, fats exhibit a comparable chemical structure. It comprises a series of interconnected carbon atoms bound to hydrogen atoms. The distinguishing factor among these fats solely pertains to the varying quantities, lengths, and configurations of hydrogen and carbon atoms within each of them.

Prior to delving into the benefits of wholesome fats, it is important to first discuss the detrimental effects of unhealthy fats. Trans fat is widely regarded as the most detrimental form of dietary fat. This adipose substance is formed through the hydrogenation process, where unsaturated oils are converted into solids to hinder their susceptibility to spoilage. This particular form of fat offers no advantageous properties to one's overall well-being and is also deemed unfit for consumption. Indeed, trans fat has been formally prohibited in various nations, such as the United States.

Conversely, polyunsaturated and monounsaturated fats are regarded as beneficial lipids predominantly derived from sources such as fish, seeds, nuts, and vegetables. This variety of lipid remains in a fluid state when subjected to ambient conditions.

When one indulges in the act of immersing bread into olive oil, one is engaging in the act of acquiring the essence and flavors inherent in the Mediterranean culinary tradition.

monounsaturated fat. This lipid possesses a sole carbon-carbon double bond, resulting in a reduction of two hydrogen atoms. This is the rationale behind the fact that monounsaturated fats retain their liquid state when exposed to ambient temperatures. Some great monounsaturated fat sources include sunflower oils, nuts, avocados, peanut oil, and olive oil.

10. Ingest Fresh Poultry, Meat, and Whole Eggs

As previously stated, meat and poultry serve as excellent protein sources, particularly for individuals following a Pegan dietary approach. They also comprise a plethora of vital nutrients, such as essential fatty acids, vitamins, zinc, iron, and iodine, which are imperative for the proper functioning of your body. Hence, it is advisable to incorporate poultry, meat, and eggs into one's dietary regimen when following a Pegan eating plan. Nevertheless, it is advisable to adhere to lean and unprocessed meat selections in order to prevent the consumption of excessive amounts of saturated fat and sodium.

Eating clean is a vague concept that does not entail any specific limitations in terms of calories or nutrition. Although delineating the precise characteristics of clean eating encompassing whole eggs, meat, and poultry may prove challenging, a prevailing commonality emerges: the conscious avoidance of packaged and processed food items that contain artificial components, excessive salt, and sugar. In this manner, you will opt for unprocessed or authentic animal-based foods rather than refined alternatives.

It is advisable to purchase whole eggs, poultry, and red meat in their freshest state, ensuring they are devoid of any synthetic additives and remain unseasoned. Inherent to their composition, these products exhibit a high nutritional density, significant protein content, and a low fat content.

After confirming the cleanliness of the purchased meat, the act of cooking will effectively eradicate any bacteria and other microorganisms. In addition to promoting good health, it will also serve as a safeguard against the occurrence of foodborne illnesses for both you and your family.

The observance of secure culinary techniques will be contingent upon the specific meat variety being prepared. Certain poultry or meat products necessitate thorough cooking, indicated by the clear flow of juices and the absence of any red or pink matter when the meat is sliced. "There are several categories of meat and poultry that necessitate thorough cooking, such as:

Prepared meat rolls

Kebabs

Sausages and rissoles

Offal (including the liver)

Pork

Various forms of avian meat, encompassing fowl such as geese, ducks, turkeys, and chickens.

Nonetheless, there exist varieties of meats that can be consumed when cooked to a rare or pink state in the center. Some of them include:

Roasting cuts

Cutlets

Steaks

The cleanliness of cooking will be contingent upon the caliber and dimensions of the meat portion. Hence, it is imperative to prioritize diligent monitoring of the temperature, rather than focusing primarily on the duration of the cooking process.

In the following section, you will discover the nutritional characteristics of both vegetarian and Paleo diets, along with the numerous advantages they offer.

consolidated Pegan diet. Pegan cuisine provides you with the most basic and nutritious elements of these two powerful dietary approaches, as well as numerous health benefits encompassing enhanced well-being, disease prevention, inflammation reduction, and increased energy levels. In addition to the numerous benefits associated with a Pegan diet, it is

Similarly, highly adaptable and easy to incorporate into your daily routine. You do not encounter difficulty in seeking out ingredients or employing novel culinary tools or methods. We ought to consistently assess the methods by which this way of life can enhance your overall well-being and success.

The Vegan Diet

The plant-based diet omits the consumption of animal-derived products, such as dairy and eggs. Vegetarianism, in essence, encompasses an entire way of life characterized by conscientiously minimizing harm to sentient animals. Ethical vegans not only banish all animal products from their diets; they also eliminate the use of animal-derived products in their daily lives. Products derived from animals or obtained by exploiting animals in any form, such as leather, wool, silk, pearls, and beeswax, are not compatible with the vegan lifestyle. Due to the dietary choices of vegans, individuals who adhere to a morally conscious vegetarian diet consume a well-structured regimen that is rich in fiber, low in saturated fat, and promotes extensive consumption of plant-based foods. Moreover, Cholesterol is not consumed in its entirety. Cholesterol, a sterol synthesized by the liver and found within cellular structures, is ubiquitous in all animal organisms. While the waxy substance remains essential, the body consistently supplies all necessary elements for its proper functioning. The excessive intake of cholesterol can be detrimental due to its tendency to promote the formation of plaque within the walls of the blood vessels, resulting in increased strain on the cardiovascular system as it strives to maintain blood flow.

Research indicates that individuals who adhere to a vegetarian diet demonstrate a reduced susceptibility to some of the most significant medical conditions, such as type 2 diabetes, cardiovascular disease, obesity, and certain forms of cancer, potentially due to the absence of cholesterol in their dietary choices.

The contemporary affluent society has recognized these advantages, resulting in the emergence of a novel manifestation of veganism: the adoption of vegan diet for reasons related to prosperity. Individuals who choose to adhere to a plant-based diet typically adhere to similar dietary principles, namely the exclusion of meat, dairy, eggs, and the use of minimal animal-derived ingredients. However, their main motivation lies in the advancement of their well-being and the reduction of their susceptibility to illness.

What dietary options are available to individuals adhering to a vegan lifestyle?

In spite of prevalent rationale, those who adhere to a vegan lifestyle have the ability to stock their refrigerators and storerooms with an extensive range of food options. Pasta, soup, tortillas, oats, bagels, potato chips, and wafers represent a fraction of the conventional food options available to individuals who adhere to a vegetarian lifestyle. Furthermore, an increasingly growing number of organizations are producing appealing vegan products.

The process of determining whether something is vegan is notably straightforward. Please inquire, "Can we ascertain if this originated from a sentient being?" If the response is affirmative, then it can be concluded that it is not suitable for a vegan diet.

Could a discussion be initiated regarding the topic of fish?

Is fish derived from a living organism? Fish, lobsters, and shrimp belong to the category of living organisms, thereby rendering fish incompatible with a vegetarian diet.

What can be inferred regarding the properties of Nectar?

Is nectar derived from a living organism? Nectar is produced by honey bees, which are living organisms; therefore, nectar is not suitable for a vegetarian diet.

Is it not imperative to address the matter regarding gelatin?

Is gelatin derived from a living organism? Gelatin is derived from the tissues of bones, ligaments, and animal skin, which renders it unsuitable for consumption by vegetarians.

Therefore, any animal-derived products are strictly forbidden within the vegan dietary guidelines. It is readily understandable to abstain from consuming a cheeseburger, macaroni, cheddar, or an omelet, and similarly straightforward to grasp that dishes comprised of leafy greens, spaghetti with marinara, and tofu over rice unequivocally belong to the category of approved options. Nevertheless, matters become uncertain when attempting to discern suitable culinary offerings - boxed, canned, and pre-packaged meals. Examining food labels is essential when adhering to a vegetarian or vegan lifestyle. In

In any situation, it is imperative that individuals, regardless of their dietary restrictions, cultivate an inclination for acquiring knowledge of nomenclature, should they find themselves uncertain or unsure. It is essential to comprehend the physiological occurrences within your body.

What are the primary sources of protein for individuals following a vegan diet?

One of the most common questions that individuals who follow a vegetarian diet often receive is, "Where do you obtain your protein?" Protein can be sourced from a variety of plant-based foods, including meat and animal-derived products. All typical dietary assortments comprise protein in varying proportions, encompassing regular items, vegetables, grains, legumes, nuts, and seeds. Incorporated within this comprehensive list are plant-based protein sources such as lentils, couscous, tofu, tempeh, quinoa, peanuts, sunflower seeds, cereal, almonds, whole wheat bread, dark beans, chickpeas, corn, peas, avocado, spinach, flaxseed, broccoli, brown rice, seitan, edamame, great northern beans, chia seeds, and artichokes.

What are the drawbacks associated with adhering to a vegan dietary regimen?

Adopting a vegan diet entails the exclusion of all animal-based products, relying instead on grains and vegetables as sources of essential protein. Therefore, the plant-based diet is frequently deficient in specific essential nutrients such as protein, calcium, vitamin B12, folate, and omega-3 fatty acids. The Pegan diet allows for the consumption of conventionally raised animal products, mitigating the potential for food insecurity. A diverse range of individuals consume refined carbohydrates as part of their vegetarian diet, such as whole wheat bread, refined white pasta, and processed white sugar. In adherence to the principles of veganism, the consumption of certain food items that are explicitly derived from animal sources is strictly avoided. However, it is worth noting that the vegan diet does allow for the inclusion of alternative sweeteners, processed oils, and refined food products which do not involve animal origin. These highly volatile food varieties are significantly contraindicated on the Pegan diet due to their association with obesity and disease.

The Paleo Diet

The Paleo diet, also known as the Old Stone Age diet, advocates for the consumption of food sources that were consumed during the Paleolithic era, spanning from the beginning of human existence (approximately 2.5 million years ago) until around 12,000 B.C.E. The Paleolithic people were hunter-gatherers, whose diet primarily consisted of natural items such as meats, poultry, fish, insects, eggs, salads, fruits, berries, nuts, and seeds.

The contemporary adherent of the Paleo lifestyle recognizes the profoundly ancestral pre-agricultural diet as that of his or her ancient predecessors. The Paleo diet is abundant in food varieties that can be hunted and gathered, akin to the lifestyle of prehistoric hunters. Clearly, those

Individuals adhering to a Paleo diet need not venture into natural environments such as forests, fields, and streams within contemporary society in order to procure their sustenance. It is solely a matter of comprehending the customs associated with unrefined culinary options.

The Paleo diet has experienced a surge in popularity, as individuals strive to adopt a healthier way of life. Given the avoidance of processed food sources and refined sugars, as well as the depletion of dairy and carbohydrates, this diet is employed with the objective of promoting a lean physique in individuals who already possess a strong body composition. Furthermore, it is widely recognized that following the Paleo lifestyle confers numerous health benefits, such as heightened levels of energy and a decreased susceptibility to conditions such as diabetes, coronary artery disease, obesity, and cancer.

What dietary options are available for individuals adhering to the paleolithic diet?

The people of the Paleolithic era sustained themselves through foraging and consumed only natural foods. Persisting in an exceedingly frivolous manner out of necessity, they embarked upon the pursuit and consolidation of their culinary selections, subsequently preparing them atop a hearth. In order to determine if something is Paleo, one must simply assess whether it aligns with the dietary preferences of early humans. The current Paleo diet places a predominant emphasis on incorporating novel varieties of meat, vegetables, and natural products into one's dietary regime. The crucial aspect is to maintain a focus on the fundamental aspect, and exclusively consume food selections that originate directly from nature, without any form of processing or artificial ingredients.

Food items that should be strictly avoided when adhering to the Paleo lifestyle include those containing artificial additives, including dairy products, grains, legumes, and starchy vegetables. No milk or cheddar. No bread or bagels. Please refrain from including beans, peanuts, peas, or soy in your selection. Additionally, adhering to the Paleo diet implies abstaining from consuming refined sugars and refined vegetable oils.

What are the sources of protein in the paleolithic diet?

It is convenient to ascertain the protein sources of individuals adhering to the Paleo diet: primarily obtained from animal-derived sources. Meat holds a significant place within the foundations of the Paleo lifestyle. In an ideal scenario, Paleo meats consist of either conventionally raised and grass-fed animals or wild game. Notwithstanding the undeniable fact that meat constitutes a substantial portion of the diet, it is advised that one refrains from consuming meats that are high in fat content, as lean meats are considered preferable. Fish, poultry, and eggs are equally deserving of consideration.

What are the drawbacks associated with following the principles of the Paleo diet?

Because of its heavy reliance on animal protein, adhering to the Paleo diet can prove challenging for individuals who follow a vegetarian or vegan lifestyle. In a comparable manner, the Paleo diet grants individuals nearly complete freedom to indulge in meat, while conveniently disregarding the importance of vegetables.

Additionally, it should be noted that the consumption of fiber-containing foods such as grains, potatoes, and beans is limited to the highest extent on this particular diet. This could potentially stimulate a decreased affirmation of dietary fiber, a crucial element for maintaining gastrointestinal health.

Similarly, the Paleo diet is inherently restrictive and may prove challenging to adhere to throughout the day, particularly when traveling or dining outside of one's home. The Pegan diet incorporates elements of both the Paleo-diet and other food sources approved by it, such as potatoes, gluten-free grains, legumes, and non-genetically modified forms of soy. This consideration towards holistic structuring and adaptability renders the Pegan diet a highly viable option for those seeking a sustainable transformation in their long-term lifestyle.

Optimal Fusion: The Pegan Diet

To propel the clinical benefits of both the veggie-darling eating routine and Paleo thins down, the Pegan diet highlights entire, authentic food assortments that are regular. Food sources originating from a receptacle do not qualify as Pegan compliant. Indeed, a significant proportion of the food items you intend to buy will not be labeled with their corresponding names.

It is highly probable that you will ultimately experience the repercussions of the Dinnermarket's deceitful practices. This dietary regimen promotes the selection of ethically sourced, organic, and humanely raised sustenance. Throughout your Pegan endeavor, it is advisable to commence your exploration of nearby farmers' commercial districts or patronize upscale markets offering a wider array of organic produce options.

This is a common occurrence wherein individuals broaden their culinary preferences and venture beyond their usual comfort zones, thereby enhancing their appreciation for diverse and high-quality food choices. The Pegan diet promotes optimal wellness through the reduction of inflammation and the regulation of blood sugar levels. It is widely recognized that this way of life confers numerous health benefits, such as weight reduction, increased stamina, and decreased susceptibility to conditions such as diabetes, cardiovascular disease, obesity, and cancer.

Is It Worth Exploring The Pegan Diet?

The pegan diet possesses certain advantages; however, it is recommended to seek guidance from a healthcare professional before embarking on this dietary approach. "Exercise prudence whenever a dietary regimen excludes entire food groups," Lembro James advises. The pegan diet may not be appropriate for individuals with health conditions such as iron or B12 deficiency. In the event that you are diagnosed with osteoporosis, it is advisable to consult with your healthcare provider in order to obtain the necessary dosage of vitamin D and calcium for optimal bone health."

If your objective is to reduce your expenditures on groceries, adhering to a rigid pegan diet may not prove to be advantageous. Organic and grass-fed meats are significantly more expensive compared to non-organic alternatives.

Furthermore, the absence of beans or legumes results in the deprivation of a cost-effective and vegetarian-friendly protein source.

You need not fully embrace the principles of the pagan lifestyle in order to acquire certain advantages from it. According to Lembo James, consuming a greater quantity of fruits and vegetables has the potential to reduce one's susceptibility to heart attacks, strokes, and cancer. However, it is important to consult your physician or nutrition specialist before disregarding the inclusion of dairy, legumes, and whole grains in your diet.

SAMPLE MENU

The pegan diet places a strong emphasis on the consumption of vegetables, while also incorporating ethically sourced meats, fish, nuts, and seeds. Certain legumes and gluten-free grains may be utilized in moderation.

Presented is an exemplar menu encompassing one week of nutritious offerings aligned with the prescribed diet plan.

MONDAY

• Morning meal option: A vegetable omelet accompanied by a plain green salad drizzled with olive oil.

• Midday meal: A salad composed of kale, chickpeas, strawberries, and avocado

• Dinner: Pan-seared wild salmon patties accompanied by oven-roasted carrots, steamed broccoli, and a light lemon vinaigrette.

TUESDAY

• Morning meal: Sweet potato "toast" accompanied by sliced avocado, pumpkin seeds, and lemon vinaigrette.

• Lunch: A bento box consisting of boiled eggs, sliced turkey, fresh vegetable sticks, fermented pickles, and blackberries.

- Dinner: Vegetable stir-fry incorporating cashews, onions, bell peppers, tomatoes, and black beans.

WEDNESDAY

- Morning meal: A blended concoction consisting of apple, kale, almond butter, and hemp seeds.

- Lunch: Remaining vegetable stir-fry.

- Dinner: Grilled shrimp and vegetable skewers accompanied by black rice pilaf

THURSDAY

- Morning meal: A pudding made with coconut and chia seeds, topped with walnuts and freshly-picked blueberries.

- For lunch, enjoy a combination of fresh greens, ripe avocado, crisp cucumber, grilled chicken, all dressed in a flavorful cider vinaigrette.

- Evening Meal: Roasted beet salad featuring pumpkin seeds, Brussels sprouts, and sliced almonds.

FRIDAY

• Morning meal: Eggs prepared in a fried manner, accompanied by kimchi and braised greens.

• Lunch: A stew consisting of lentils and vegetables, accompanied by a serving of sliced cantaloupe

• Dinner: A salad consisting of radishes, jicama, guacamole, and grass-fed beef strips.

SATURDAY

• Breakfast: A nutritious morning meal comprising of a bowl of overnight oats prepared with cashew milk, chia seeds, walnuts, and a medley of berries.

• Noon Meal: Remnants of lentil and vegetable stew

• Dinner: Roast pork loin accompanied by steamed vegetables, leafy greens, and quinoa.

SUNDAY

- Morning meal: Vegetable omelet served with a basic green salad

• Midday meal: Salad rolls prepared in the style of Thai cuisine, served with a cashew cream sauce and slices of orange.

• Dinner: Remaining pork loin and vegetables

Note

The pegan diet places emphasis on a diet rich in vegetables, along with the inclusion of protein, wholesome fats, and select fruits. Grains and legumes are encompassed, albeit with lower regularity.

CONCLUTION

Although there is no requirement to limit calorie intake or adhere to strict meal timing, it is worth noting that by adopting a pegan diet, one may inadvertently overlook crucial nutritional elements that are found in essential foods such as whole grains, dairy, and legumes. If you are in search of a dietary regimen that effectively mitigates inflammation and fosters optimum well-being, it is worth contemplating other discerningly composed eating plans such as the flexitarian diet or Mediterranean diet.

Please keep in mind that adhering to either a prolonged or brief dietary regimen may not be essential for your specific situation, as numerous diets available often prove ineffective, particularly over an extended duration. While we abstain from endorsing fad diet trends or unsustainable weight loss methods, we provide factual information to empower you in making an informed decision that aligns with your nutritional requirements, genetic predisposition, financial constraints, and objectives.

If your objective entails achieving weight reduction, it is crucial to bear in mind that shedding pounds does not automatically equate to embodying optimal health. Furthermore, there exist numerous alternative avenues through which to pursue overall well-being. Physical activity, adequate rest, and various lifestyle elements significantly contribute to one's holistic well-being. The optimal diet is always the one that is well-rounded and suits your lifestyle.

Lactose-Free Crepes

3 eggs

3 teaspoons of extra virgin olive oil

Salt to taste.

600 ml Almond (almond milk)

100g 00 flour

100 g oatmeal

50 g cornstarch

Transfer unbroken eggs into a spacious bowl. Crack the eggs with a whisk and delicately combine the yolk with the egg whites (as demonstrated in the video, the eggs have already been cracked and placed in a bowl). Transfer the eggs into a receptacle and incorporate a small amount of salt. Incorporate the strained 00 flour into the mixture and combine it with the eggs using a whisk. Add a small amount of Mandorla Drink Bio and continue blending using a whisk. Incorporate the oatmeal and cornstarch into the mixture by sifting through both ingredients. Incorporate the Mandorla Drink Bio gradually, vigorously whisking it into the mixture. Add a small amount of salt and three teaspoons of extra virgin olive oil.

Continue to exert strong pressure while kneading the dough to avoid the formation of any lumps. Allow the dough to undergo a period of rest in the refrigerator for a minimum duration of one hour. Prepare the dish by utilizing a crepe maker or a low-edged non-stick frying pan. Place a scoop of the dough in the middle of the heated pan and lightly coat it with a drizzle of extra virgin olive oil. Swivel the pan while maintaining a slight inclination, ensuring the even distribution of the dough across the entirety of the base. Return it to the stovetop over a gentle flame until the crepes have cooked sufficiently to release from the surface. Flip it and proceed with cooking for a few moments more. After the preparations are complete, proceed to fill as per your preference.

Green Curry Mushrooms

Ingredients:

.

.¼ teaspoon salt

.1 cup soy milk

.1 tablespoon green curry paste

1 1/2 cups water

.1 1/2 tablespoons vegetable oil

.1 cup mushrooms, drained and cubed

Directions:

1. Choose the Sauté function on the Instant Pot. Upon reaching the desired temperature, promptly introduce vegetable oil into the heated Instant Pot. Mix in mushrooms. Periodically combine

the ingredients and cook for approximately 5 minutes, until evenly browned and delicately caramelized. Season with salt.

2. Incorporate soy milk into the green curry paste.

3. Please ensure that the lid is securely fastened onto the pot. Please ensure the closure of the tension delivery valve. Please choose the "Manual" setting and adjust the pressure cooker to operate at High Pressure for a duration of 5 minutes. Upon completion of the designated cooking duration, it is advised to refrain from agitating the pot for a duration of 10 minutes, followed by the subsequent release of any pressure that may still be present.

Homemade Falafel

Ingredients

- 1.5 tbsps. freshly squeezed lemon juice
- ¼ tsp. cumin
- Sea salt
- Black pepper
- 4 tbsps. oat flour
- 4 tbsps. olive
- 4 c. collard greens
- 15.5 oz. washed and drained chickpeas
- 3 chopped medium cloves garlic
- 1.5 tbsps. tahini

Instructions

Incorporate all the ingredients into the food processor, excluding the oil and oat flour, and subsequently process them until thoroughly blended.

Transfer the mixture to a bowl after thoroughly combining all the ingredients, then gradually incorporate one tablespoon of oat flour at a time until the mixture reaches the desired thickness.

Savor the flavors of the seasonings and make necessary adjustments to achieve the desired taste.

Place a frying pan on the stovetop and heat it to a medium temperature, then gradually introduce 2 tablespoons of oil with each addition. Gently agitate it to evenly distribute over the surface of the pan.

Place four falafel into the pan simultaneously.

Inspect them after a duration of 2 minutes and rotate them when they achieve a dark golden brown hue, continuing this process for approximately 4 minutes.

Continue cooking until all sides have achieved a tasteful golden brown color.

Accompany the dish with hummus and a sprinkle of paprika. Enjoy.

Ingredients

- ¼ teaspoons fresh ground black pepper
- 2 medium/ large sized avocados, halve or pitted
- 4 large whole eggs

<u>DIRECTIONS</u>

Kindly ensure that your oven is preheated to a temperature of 425 degrees Fahrenheit.

Remove a portion of the avocado flesh from each half, ensuring there is adequate room to accommodate an egg.

Gently arrange the avocado halves in a single layer inside the 8 by 8-inch baking pan, which has been conveniently lined with foil.

Carefully enclose the avocados by folding the foil around their outer edges.

Place one egg into each half of the avocado, and season them generously with black pepper.

Cook in the oven for approximately 12 to 15 minutes without a cover until you achieve the desired degree of doneness.

Extract from the oven and allow them to settle for a duration of 5 minutes.

Serve and enjoy!